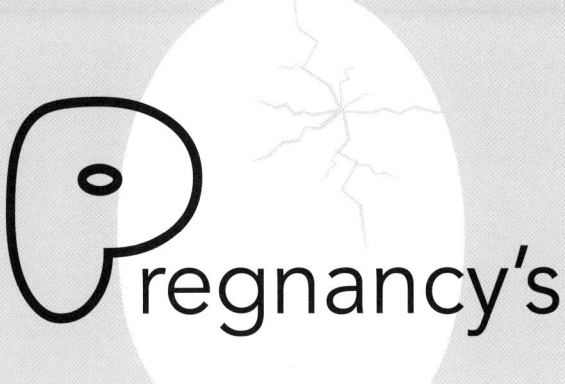

Pregnancy's

Little
Headaches

before the big day!

A division of the Quarto Publishing Group USA Inc.
276 Fifth Avenue Suite 206
New York, New York 10001

ROCK POINT and the distinctive Rock Point logo are trademarks of
the Quarto Publishing Group USA Inc.

ISBN-13: 978-1-631060-11-3

Printed in China

2 4 6 8 10 9 7 5 3 1

1

first trimester

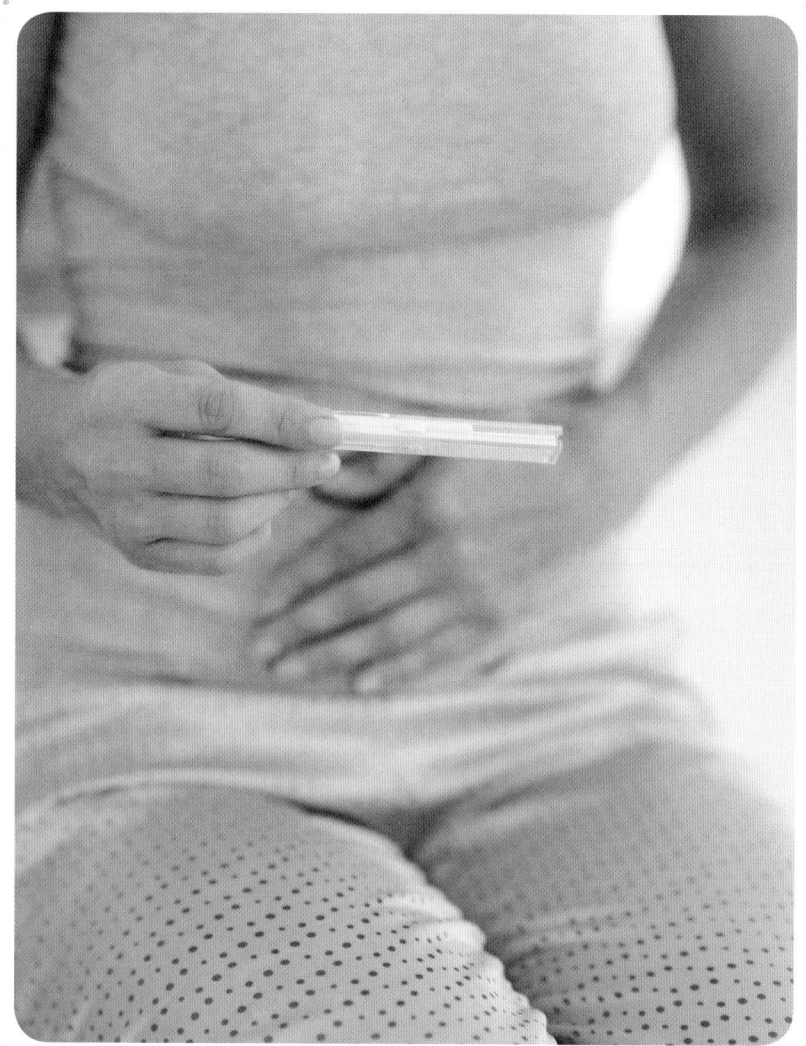

1st

trimester
little headaches

"Oh,
so that's why
I've had PMS
for FIVE WEEKS."

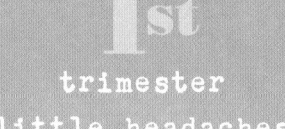

1st
trimester
little headaches

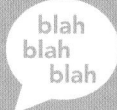

Getting really good at lying
and denying it
for the first twelve weeks.

1st

trimester
little headaches

Not giving anything away
when your best friend leans in and,
concerned, asks if you've
"gained a little weight."

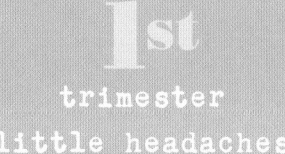

1st

Bumping into your
gossipy colleague while
standing in line at the pharmacy
trying to conceal
a home pregnancy test.

1st

Getting pregnant on your honeymoon,
and watching people
mentally count backwards
to your wedding date
as you tell them the news.

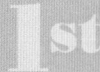

1st
trimester
little headaches

Coming up with
another credible excuse
for why you're not having that
luscious, oh-so-inviting cocktail.
Such as…

1st

- It'll clash with my Zoloft/Prozac/Valium/Flintstones vitamin.

- I'm on a solids-only diet.

- The vodka is not kosher.

- I have a colonoscopy appointment.

- I'm allergic to juniper, potatoes, all grains, and grapes.

- I'm still drunk from lunch.

- "Red? Oh, I'm only drinking white. From Argentina. "

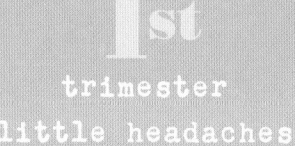

1st
trimester
little headaches

The sixth obstretrician you interviewed,
oh, he was absolutely perfect.
A shining model of skill,
compassion, and support.

And slated to be on vacation
during your delivery date.

1st
trimester
little headaches

Having morning sickness
in the afternoon,
and evening,
and always.

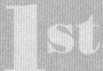

1st

trimester
little headaches

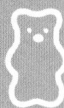

Pretending to be thrilled
at your sonogram image of—
a lima bean?
Cashew?
Gummy bear?

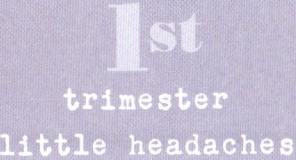

1st
trimester
little headaches

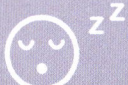

Falling asleep at work.
At the gym.
At your best friend's birthday party.
While standing up—
almost.

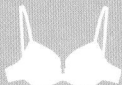

♡A♡!

You've achieved your secret wish
to have bigger breasts—

BUT

they hurt when you shower,
walk down stairs,
work out,
walk the dog.

1st

trimester
little headaches

Bathroom Breaks:

5 am—time to pee!

6:05 am—time to pee!

7:02 am—time to go!

8:17 am—again!

And thus a new daily—
and nightly—
routine emerges.

1st
trimester
little headaches

Experiencing your
FIRST vomit-free morning
when suddenly you get a whiff of:

strong perfume

meat

sushi

boiled beef . . .

1st
trimester
little headaches

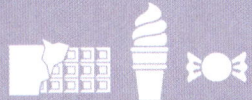

Wondering
why your cravings
never involve fruit,
lettuce, carrots,
celery . . .

1st
trimester
little headaches

Will crushed up prenatal vitamins
make a good topping for ice cream,
pizza, cupcakes,
rye bread with butter . . .

1st

trimester
little headaches

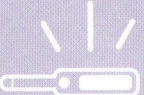

The WHOO-HOO moment:
Yeah, I AM bloated and blotchy!
Yep, my hair DOES look weird.
And I am HAPPY about it all
because . . .

I'M PREGNANT!

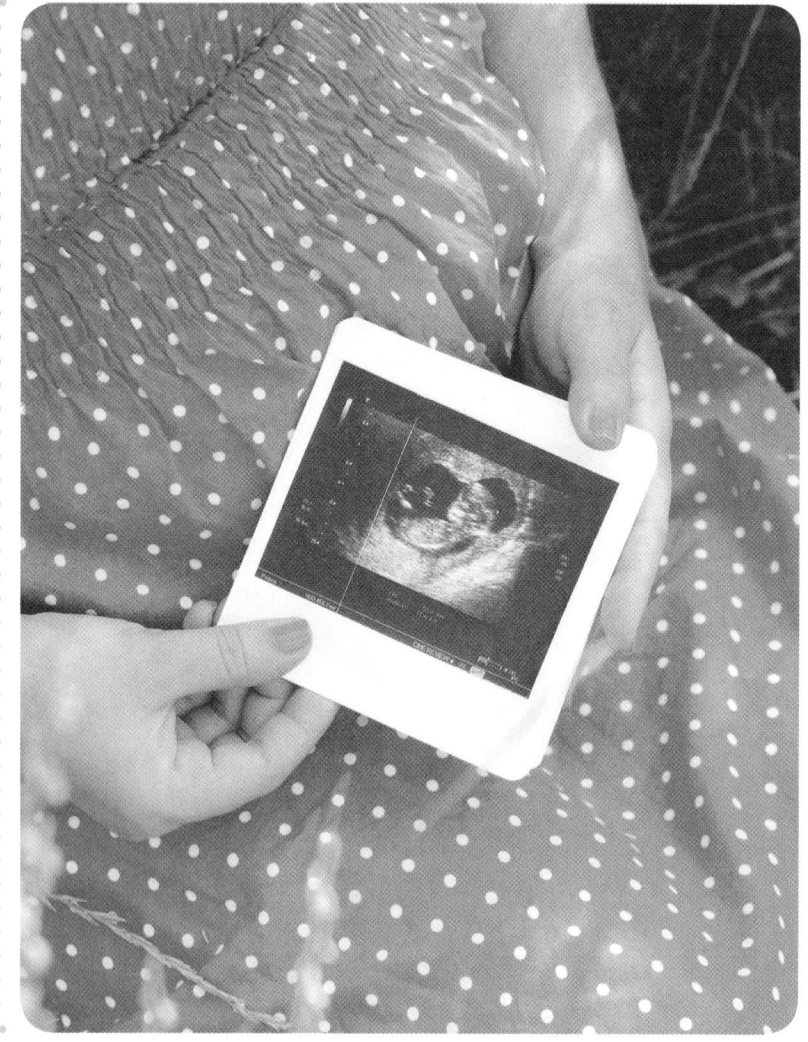

second trimester

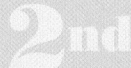

2nd

trimester

little headaches

You're coughing, itchy-eyed,
chest-and-nose congested,
running a fever,
and can take
ABSOLUTELY NOTHING
for it.

2nd

trimester

little headaches

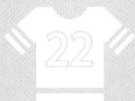

"Does my husband's XL football jersey make me look fat?"

2nd
trimester
little headaches

Accepting that
at least for the next six months
you will, and must,
hate your size-four, petite friend.

2nd

trimester
little headaches

Looking forward
to getting together with a friend
who's in the same trimester...
until you see how much smaller
her belly is.

Shopping for something formal,
flattering, and that just happens
to have an elasto-waistband
for the swanky black-tie wedding
you'll be attending.

2nd

trimester
little headaches

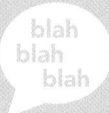

Receiving advice from everyone
who's ever had a child…
or been one!

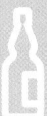

"Thanks, Grandma.
I will definitely consider giving the baby
'a wee nip of whiskey'
if he ever gets too fussy."

GREAT!

The childbirth class you want
has an opening!
A week after your due date.

Ah, the heartburn,
the indigestion,
the zits.

All part of nature's miracle.

2nd

Twenty-week sonogram gender-dilemma:

Blue? Pink?

Sheila or Sherman?

Must know! Must wait!

I want to know! He doesn't!

Better to just paint the nursery
yellow or green?

2nd
trimester
little headaches

The Uncomfortable Equation:

30 pounds (*total weight gain so far*)
− 1 pound (*baby's weight so far*)
────────
29 pounds (*potato chips, tacos*
          all-chocolate breakfasts,
          hotdogs, cookies)

2nd

trimester
little headaches

———

**"Of course,
Person I Don't Know,
I'd be glad to discuss
my belly size
with you."**

2nd

trimester
little headaches

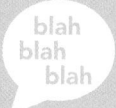

Hearing Mom's tale of your birth
for the umpteenth time:

"And as I begged your father
to let them knock me out…"

"My screams shattered, *shattered*
two of the delivery room windows."

2nd

"Of course, I refused extra fuss
just because I happened to be giving birth."

"Ninety-two hours of the most intense,
painful, mindbending…"

"And your dad? He was utterly worthless."

"So hairy! And wrinkly! And LOUD!"

"And I cooked a four-course dinner,
did three loads of laundry,
cut my own hair,
and varnished the front porch
the very next week."

2nd

trimester
little headaches

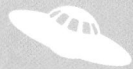

What if there really is an alien in there?

2nd
trimester
little headaches

Feeling guilty about skipping
the "strongly recommended" methods
for pre-nursing nipple-toughening.

2nd
trimester
little headaches

Can focus!
Can work out!
Can do normal stuff…
SORT OF!

2nd

trimester
little headaches

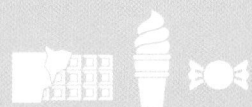

Discovery:

Stressed spelled
backwards is
DESSERTS!

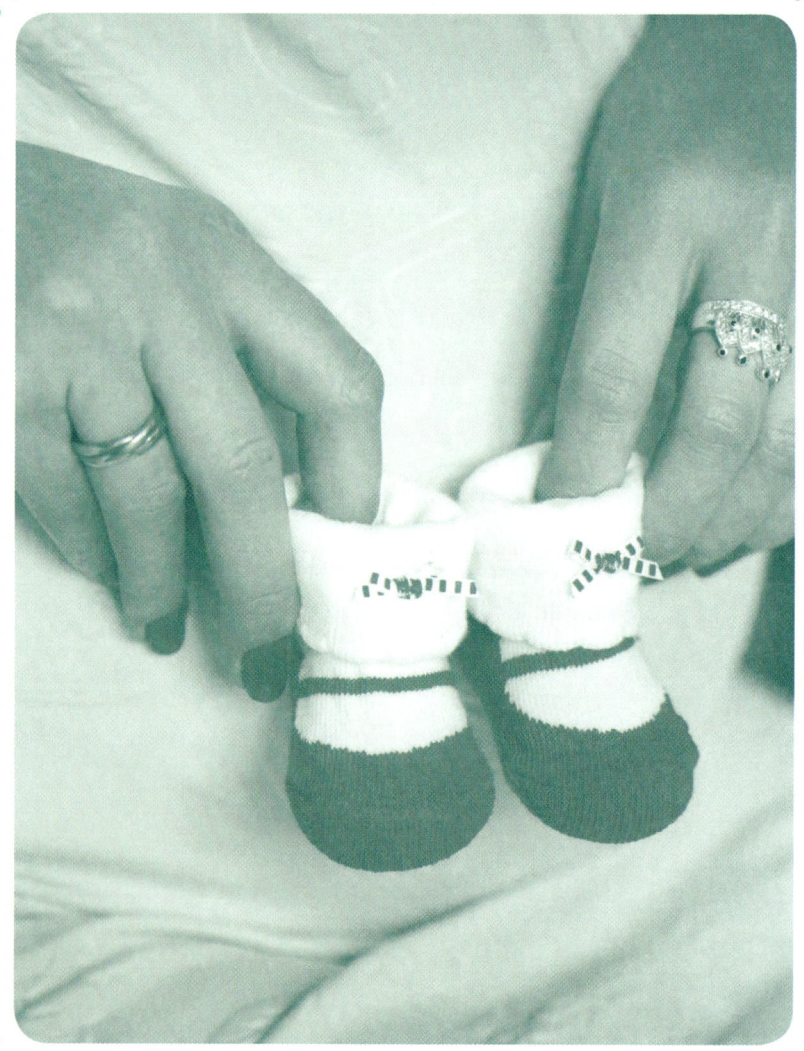

third trimester

3rd
trimester
little headaches

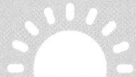

Waking up one morning
to discover that your belly button
has changed from an "innie"
to an "outtie."

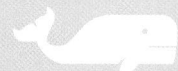

He says you look like a goddess.

You feel more
like a beached whale.

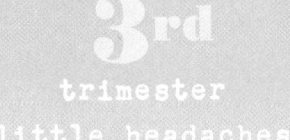

3rd
trimester
little headaches

He's signaling he's "in the mood."
You are, too!

But with the Little Invader
taking up so much real estate…

3rd
trimester
little headaches

DO NOT DISTURB

Let's just try having very quiet sex.
Maybe the baby won't notice?

3rd
trimester
little headaches

"**O**f course,
Total Stranger,
why wouldn't I want you
to touch my belly?"

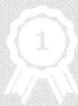

Criteria for choosing the BEST
car seat, stroller, crib:
Safest!
Most popular!
Highest rated!
Celebrity-endorsed!
Nine out of ten pediatricians recommend…!
Trendsetting!
Classic!
Innovative!
Modern mom loves…!
AGHHHHHHH!

3rd

trimester
little headaches

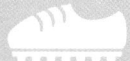

Realizing that there are no
swollen-ankle-flattering shoes.

The all-night search
for a comfortable sleeping position:
1 am—writhe.
2 am—twist.
3 am—flip.
4 am—flop.
5 am—wake him up.
Because it's his baby, too!

3rd
trimester
little headaches

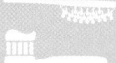

Having only enough energy
to brush your hair or teeth.
But not both.

3rd

trimester
little headaches

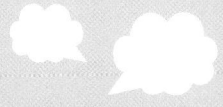

HUFF-A-PUFF!

So this is what it's like
to live 5,000 feet
above sea level!

3rd
trimester
little headaches

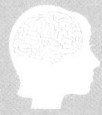

Telltale signs
that pregnancy brain has set in:

• Wondering why your TV remote
  won't open the garage door.

• Moisturizer on your toothbrush.
  Toothpaste on your face.

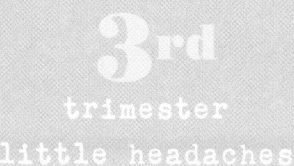

3rd
trimester
little headaches

- Finding your cellphone in the fridge.

- Forgetting the multiplication tables.
  And your work phone number.
  And your husband's middle name.
  And where you put…everything!

  - Spending an hour searching
    for the shirt
    YOU'RE WEARING.

3rd
trimester
little headaches

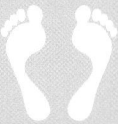

The shock when the sight line
to your feet becomes
wholly obstructed.

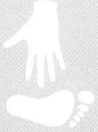

The blissful joy of
a nightly foot massage.

3rd

trimester

little headaches

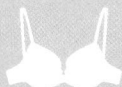

♡our first D-cup.

And double-D.

And E!

When will this
new-cup-of-the-month
madness end?

3rd

trimester
little headaches

Deciding that shaving your legs
is totally optional
and completely impossible.

At the obstetrician's office:
The person before you has just announced:
"I'm in labor.
And I'm being admitted!"

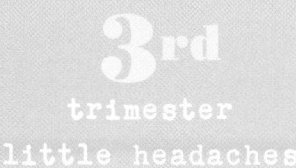

3rd
trimester
little headaches

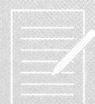

Choosing a name that...

• has zero negative associations

• will travel well
throughout his/her lifetime

• is memorable but not bizarre

• is inspiring, and flattering

• will compel everyone to love him/her

• begins with an "L," or "B",

and...

3rd

trimester
little headaches

When even your hair
feels puffy and swollen.

3rd
trimester
little headaches

Bursting into tears
when being told that
you really don't look that fat.

3rd

trimester
little headaches

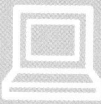

Making the mistake
of Googling the hospital
you've chosen
for your delivery
and reading EVERY
negative review.

3rd
trimester
little headaches

Wishing
work, housework,
and every annoying obligation
could just cease to exist
until after you've safely delivered
the "Most Wonderful Baby"
and completed
the "Most Joyous Maternity Leave"
EVER!

3rd
trimester
little headaches

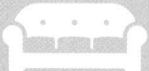

HEAVE-HO!

When you cannot leave the couch
without an assist.

3rd
trimester
little headaches

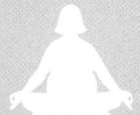

You do daily light yoga
while the baby opts
for nightly gymnastics.

3rd
trimester
little headaches

ⓟregnancy Pro:

must buy new shoes!

ⓟregnancy Con:

they are a full size larger.

3rd
trimester
little headaches

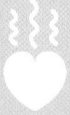

When even oatmeal and pudding
give you heartburn.

3rd

trimester
little headaches

!

Hemorrhoids...
varicose veins...
and stretch marks—

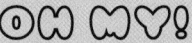

3rd

trimester
little headaches

Secretly hoping
for the most
boring delivery story ever.

Anticipating when your water breaks:
So, how much water
are we talking about?
A cup?
Quart?
Gallon?!

Should I travel with a bucket from now on?

3rd
trimester
little headaches

Wearing
"SERIOUSLY?"
in reaction to
your proud announcement
of the baby's
painstakingly chosen name.

3rd

trimester

little headaches

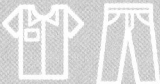

Getting really tired of wearing
your husband's shirts and jeans.

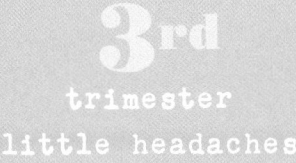

3rd
trimester
little headaches

Weekly awful labor-and-delivery stories:

"It was a dark and stormy night..."

"And as an unforecasted hurricane
swept up the driveway..."

"We ended up naming him
after the cab driver/delivery man."

"And when they refused
to give me a third epidural..."

"And then traffic came to a complete stop..."

"The engine/elevator/air conditioning/
electricity/cell phone just quit.
Completely."

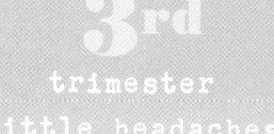

3rd
trimester
little headaches

Desperately wanting
an ironclad assurance from the doctor
that, yes, it is really, truly,
absolutely possible for
THAT
to get out of
THIS.

3rd
trimester
little headaches

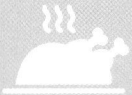

Bursting into tears at a jokey friend's
"Oh, I hear it's no more difficult
than passing a Thanksgiving turkey!"

3rd
trimester
little headaches

"♡es, I'm completely
positive it's not twins,
you *$&^#!"

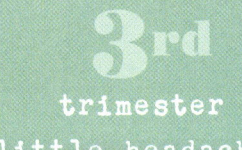

3rd
trimester
little headaches

$\mathcal{T}$he Even More Uncomforable Equation:

   45 pounds (*total weight gain so far*)

− 15 pounds (*weight of baby and afterbirth*)

   30 pounds (*chips, ice cream, breakfast pizza,*
                      midnight cookies)

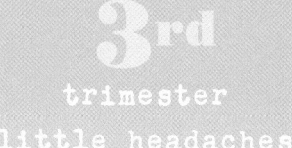

3rd
trimester
little headaches

Excellent baby shower
registry additions:

foot massages!

naps!

leg waxes!

compliments!

Secret Will-Do-It-All Assistant!

3rd
trimester
little headaches

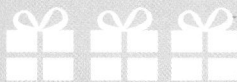

Baby shower dilemma:

Any way to avoid the cutesy
smell-the-poop games,
and still get
ALL THE STUFF?

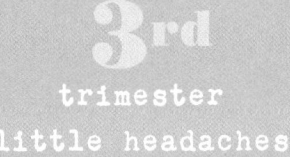

3rd
trimester
little headaches

Dreaming about not
wearing a T-shirt to the beach.

3rd
trimester
little headaches

Can't.

Button.

ANYTHING.

Plenty of room to fit
all the new baby stuff.
If we put the nursery in the garage
or under the front porch.

3rd
trimester
little headaches

False labor?
Go home and relax?
Are you kidding?

3rd
trimester
little headaches

Experiencing your day,
night, and next-day labor pains
until the…

amazing,

awesome,

astonishing,

adorable

ARRIVAL!

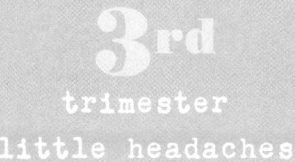

3rd

trimester
little headaches

Ouzzah!

Welcome!

Mazel tov!

Congratulations!

Job Well Done!

3rd

trimester
little headaches

Phew!